KETOGENIC DIET

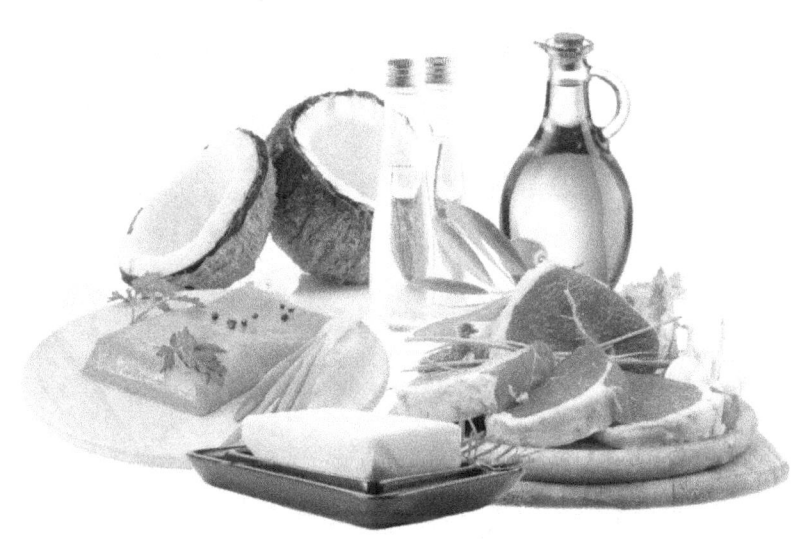

DANIEL ISACCS

TABLE OF CONTENTS

INTRODUCTION TO KETOGENIC DIET

The Ketogenic diet involves significantly reducing carbohydrate intake while increasing protein to the levels necessary to maintain muscle mass with the calorie ratios approximating 50% protein, 20% low glycemic index carbohydrates and 30% therapeutic fats.

The general dietary guidelines involve avoidance of high carbohydrate foods such as bread, pasta, potatoes, rice etc. as well as all simple carbohydrates such as sugar, honey and fruit juice.

Recent studies have demonstrated that a higher protein, low carbohydrate diet promotes superior results for fat loss, improvements in blood lipid parameters and increased thermogenesis in individuals with obesity and insulin resistance and may help to resolve the metabolic blocks that can prevent fat loss.

How does it work?

Your body normally relies on carbohydrates for energy. It breaks them down into glucose, which is your main source of fuel.

The Ketogenic diet produces very good results when followed consistently. Long term success is more likely if a holistic attitude is adopted that addresses diet, exercise, nutritional supplements and psychological factors as well as any specific health challenges that are unique to the individual.

WHAT IS A KETOGENIC DIET?

Basically, it is a diet that causes the body to enter a state of ketosis. Ketosis is a natural and healthy metabolic state in which the body burns its own stored fat (producing ketones), instead of using glucose (the sugars from carbohydrates found in the Standard American Diet - SAD).

Metabolically speaking, ketogenic foods are very powerful. The amazing benefit is that these foods are also delicious, natural whole foods that are extremely healthy for you.

So what foods are encouraged?

Some of the best-tasting, most fulfilling foods are part of this plan, including lean meats like beef and chicken, healthy sources of protein and high-quality fats like eggs, butter, olive oil, coconut oil and avocado. Also, delicious leafy-green vegetables like kale, chard, and spinach, as well as cruciferous vegetables like broccoli, cabbage and cauliflower.

These foods can be combined with seeds, nuts, sprouts, and a wide range of other amazing foods that lead to incredible health benefits that give your body the protein, healthy fats, and nutrients it needs while providing metabolism-boosting meals for easy cooking at home or on the go.

Protein is included in every meal as this helps to reduce appetite, regulate blood glucose levels and preserve lean muscle mass. Examples of protein foods are fish, chicken, turkey, meat, eggs, cheese, tofu and tempeh. Protein drinks such as whey protein isolate or soy protein may be utilized. Soy protein is especially beneficial as it has been shown to stimulate thyroid hormone production, reduce fat levels and promote fat loss, due to the phytoestrogens and essential fatty acids it contains.

Adequate fat intake is also essential as this enhances fat burning by the body while reducing synthesis of fatty acids in the body which both promote fat loss. Optimal sources of fats are flaxseed oil, fish oil, avocado, olive oil, nuts and seeds.To provide balanced nutrition, vitamins, minerals, and fiber and to promote detoxification it is also essential to consume 3-4 cups of low carbohydrate vegetables or salad daily with one optional serve of fresh fruit daily.

When beginning a Ketogenic diet program some discomfort may be experienced such as headaches, irritability, fatigue and hunger for the first 2-7 days, however thereafter it is very easy to adhere to the diet and it actually reduces appetite, carbohydrate cravings and increases energy levels.

A typical day on the Ketogenic diet may be as follows:

Breakfast:

Scrambled eggs or tofu with parsley, scallions, spinach and tomato OR

Protein powder blended with fresh or frozen berries

Lunch:

Salad with tuna/salmon/eggs/cottage cheese

Dinner:

Fish, chicken, turkey, tofu or meat with steamed or stir fried low carbohydrate vegetables

Snacks: (2-3 daily)

Protein drink OR

Hard boiled egg OR

Handful of nuts or seeds

When the ideal body fat percentage is achieved the diet may be gradually adjusted to include more complex carbohydrates such as whole grains, starchy vegetables and fruit while as much as possible avoiding all other simple carbohydrates such as sugar, honey and refined flours. Simultaneously it is essential to ensure that protein is included in every meal.

This more relaxed type of dietary approach can be maintained indefinitely in conjunction with a regular exercise program to ensure that body weight and composition remains stable.

Tips for Success on the Ketogenic Diet

1.) Drink tons of water.

While on a ketogenic diet, your body has a hard time retaining as much water as it needs, so staying properly hydrated is absolutely essential. Many experts recommend that men intake a minimum of 3 liters of beverages each day, while the figure for women is 2.2 liters daily. A good indicator of proper hydration is the color of your urine. If your urine is clear or light yellow, you're most likely properly hydrated. Keep a bottle of water with you everywhere you go!

2.) Don't forget the fat!

Simply put, our bodies need fuel to function. When we limit our carbohydrate intake, especially to levels that induce ketosis, our bodies need an alternate fuel source. Since protein is not an efficient source of energy, our bodies turn to fat. Any fat you eat while in ketosis is used for energy, making it very difficult to store fat while in ketosis. Choose healthy, unsaturated fats as often as possible: foods like avocados, olives, nuts, and seeds are ideal.

3.) Find your carb limit.

All of our bodies are different. Some dieters will need to adhere to a strict low-carbohydrate diet that entails consuming less than 20 grams per day of carbs. Other dieters will find that they can comfortably stay in ketosis while consuming 50, 75, or 100 grams of carbohydrates. The only way to know for sure is trial and error. Purchase Ketostix or any brand of ketone urinalysis strips and find out your carbohydrate limit. If you find that you have a bit of wiggle room, it will make sticking to your diet that much easier.

4.) Be smart about liquor.

One of the great aspects of the ketogenic diet is that you can drink liquor while on it without throwing your weight loss too far off course. You can drink unsweetened liquors like vodka, rum, tequila, gin, whiskey, scotch, cognac, and brandy, along with the occasional low-carb beer. Use low-carb mixers and drink plenty of water to stay hydrated, as hangovers are notoriously bad while in ketosis. And remember, calories still count, so don't go overboard. All things in moderation.

5.) Be patient.

While the ketogenic diet is known for rapid weight loss, especially in the early stages of the diet, weight loss is always a slow, time-consuming process. Don't freak out if the scale doesn't show weight loss, or shows slight weight increases, for a few days. Your weight varies day-to-day (and throughout the day) based upon a number of factors. Don't forget to use metrics like how your clothes fit or body measurements to see progress beyond what the scale shows.

WHY SHOULD YOU DO A KETOGENIC DIET?

A Ketogenic Diet is high in fat, low in carbohydrate, protein-filled plan that makes the body burn fat as opposed to carbohydrates.

Though it has been used to treat epilepsy in children, it is also a popular weight loss and core strengthening diet.

Based off the proven 4:1 ratio, the secret of the plan is to consume four fats for every one carbohydrate or protein.

Below are seven reasons why a Ketogenic Diet could be right for you.

1. Ketogenic Diets and the Treatment of Diseases

Though used primarily to treat epilepsy, studies show that a reduction in intake of carbohydrates can drastically boost your metabolism, leading not only to weight loss, but in some cases, in the amelioration or the elimination of disease.

Ketogenic diets have been shown to help with Cardiovascular diseases as well, by lowering cholesterol and by pumping up blood lipid panels.

A Ketogenic diet has also been proven to help with Type Two Diabetes by lowering insulin resistance and reduced glucose outputs.

2. Lowering Carb Intake To Fight Obesity

A second study shows that adopting a Ketogenic diet can significantly help with weight loss by reducing the BMI of patients.

As obesity becomes a worldwide problem that affected millions, the benefits of exercise alone are not enough to lose weight.

The study found that a Ketogenic Diet not only lowered cholesterol and blood glucose, as above, but that it also specifically lowered the level of triglycerides, a major factor in weight gain.

Additionally, once patients went off the diet and returned to one high in carbohydrates, they almost immediately gained back the weight.

3. Low-carb Brain Fuel

One of the most important factors regarding the Ketogenic diet is the benefits it has on the human brain.

By increasing the body's circulation of ketones, better and stronger fuel is pumped into the brain, leading to not only an increase in focus and energy, but also acting as a kind of prevention and treatment for a multitude of neurological disorders.

4. Eliminating Glucose To Force The Body To Burn Fat

The goal of the Ketogenic diet is to force our bodies to enter Ketosis, which means that instead of relying on glucose, created by the breaking down of carbohydrates, to fuel ourselves throughout the day, the body must instead look to using stored fat to energize the mind and body.

When the necessary amount of carbohydrates needed to convert into energy are restricted, the body find those materials from other sources.

An entirely new method of metabolism is created, and serves as a jump-start for weight loss. While it is important to remember to work out while on a Ketogenic diet, it has been proven to be far more beneficial than simply exercise alone.

5. Ketogenic Diets and Their Effects on Cellular Energy

This study also points toward an important factor in the success of the ketogenic diet — its impact on cells in the body.

Since we already know that an increased circulation of ketones provides more brain energy, that means that the ketones could also lead to an increase in the number of brain cells themselves.

Additionally, these new and improved brain cells also contain the mitochondria, the powerhouse of the cells, that are packed with higher levels of energy and an increase in productivity thanks to the ketones.

This leads to increased levels of energy and feelings of alertness, which may also be responsible for an increase in metabolic production and the burning of stored fat.

Because of these factors, the Ketogenic Diet has also been shown to improve brain function and to help with memory loss.

6. The Ketogenic Diet Can Potentially Protect Against Cancer

Though there are no guarantees that adopting a Ketogenic diet will prevent cancer, studies have shown that, again due to the increased brain function it provides, the Ketogenic diet has been effective, when used in conjunction with medication, in reduces cancerous brain tumors.

Also, when used in addition to radiation therapy, the Ketogenic diet has eradicated brain tumor cells.

It is thought that the success of the diet in terms of aiding patients with tumors and cancers is due to the diet's limitation of growth factor stimulation — which, of course, means that it could limit or halt the growth of a tumor.

It may also help to cut back on inflammation surrounding the area of the tumor, which could lead to a reduction in both pain and the size of the tumor itself.

Though it is important to once again stress that a Ketogenic diet cannot on its own protect against cancer and completely eliminate tumors already within the human body, it has been shown, when used in conjunction with other treatments, to speed the recovery process, reduce pain, and help to decrease the size of cancerous and malign tumors.

7. The Power of Antioxidants

Since the Ketogenic diet is also high in antioxidants, studies have shown that it prevents oxidative damage, which can occur during hypoglycemia.

The diet prevents the destruction of weaker cells in addition to creating newer, stronger ones to fight off infection and disease.

An increase in antioxidants within the body can help to balance out the amount of free radicals within the body, which, when out of balance, can lead to decreased energy and a reduced immune system.

When free radicals are removed from the bloodstream, not only is the immune system boosted, but memory function improves, muscles in the eyes are strengthened, and even mood and memory issues are greatly ameliorated.

Final Thoughts

Though the Ketogenic diet has been in place for hundreds of years as a means to treat disease, its proven success in recent studies has lead to a resurgence of the diet.

When combined with exercise, adopting a Ketogenic diet can lead to dramatic and long-term success.

By improving brain function, forcing the body to burn fat and find new ways of creating energy, lowering the intake of carbohydrates, and upping the intake of fat into the body, the Ketogenic diet has a multitude of benefits, and is safe for almost anyone to undertake.

THE BENEFITS OF A KETOGENIC DIET

1. Weight Loss

Low carb, high fat diets have been used for centuries by doctors when working with obese patients.

Many people successfully use ketogenic diets today in their quest for decreased body fat levels for these exact reasons. By consuming a higher fat/lower carb diet you also retrain the body to use fat as an energy source. This allows the body to tap into its own fat reserves – burning it as energy. If your body is used to burning carbohydrates for fuel, then when those carb sources run out or are not consumed, your body craves another 'hit'. Despite there being a plentiful store of fat mass.

2. Anti-aging

Lowering oxidative stress in the body is one way to increase lifespan. It seems that by lowering insulin levels, oxidative stress in turn is decreased. A ketogenic diet decreases insulin levels – allowing the formation of ketones to be used as fuel.

3. Lower Blood Sugar (Type 2 Diabetes)

Speaking of lowered insulin levels, a result of running off ketones allows an individual to control, and lower, their blood sugar levels. The ability to utilise fat and ketones as fuel for the body mean a pre-diabetic or even a type 2 diabetic, no longer has to worry about excess blood sugar levels and the need to source exogenous insulin.

4. Cardiovascular Disease and Metabolic Syndrome

Researchers found that the contributors to heart disease (evaluated blood sugar, high blood triglycerides, low HDL cholesterol, high blood pressure etc) are improved when following a low carb, ketogenic type diet.

5. Polycystic Ovary Syndrome (PCOS)

PCOS often occurs along with insulin resistance causing a range of hormonal issues in woman including infertility.

A ketogenic diet – due to its extremely low carb intake – can help address insulin resistance and in turn help with suffers of PCOS. In fact, a pilot study has concluded that a ketogenic diet led to a significant improvement in body weight, fasting insulin, testosterone markets and LH/FSH ratio in woman with PCOS. Two woman even became pregnant during the study.

6. Brain Function

Other than fat loss, a big reason why so many people rave about ketogenic diets is due to improved brain function, clarity of thought, memory recall, improved learning etc. etc.

Ketogenic diets, even in the short term, can improve memory function in older adults. Also, a ketogenic diet was shown to increase ATP concentrations and the number of hippocampal mitochondria in the brain of mice by up to 50%. The hippocampus is involved in memory, learning and emotion.

7. Irritable Bowel Syndrome (IBS)

Many who suffer from IBS (chronic diarrhoea, stomach discomfort, bloating etc.) would probably shudder at the thought of eating a high fat low carb diet. Upping fat intake can lead to increased diarrhoea at first, but it's the long term effects of a ketogenic diet that are appealing to those suffering from IBS.

Numerous studies have found that low sugar consumption can assist with IBS symptoms and one particular study found that a ketogenic diet provides adequate relief, and improves abdominal pain, stool habits, and quality of life in individuals suffering from IBS.

8. Increased Mitochondrial Function

Mitochondria are our cells energy factories, without mitochondria in our cells we would be dead. A lot of our health, energy, sports performance, immune function etc is dependent upon how well our mitochondria are functioning.

The mitochondria – work much better on a ketogenic diet as they are able to increase energy levels in a stable, long-burning, efficient, and steady way. Not only that, a ketogenic diet induces epigenetic changes which increases the energetic output of our mitochondria, reduces the production of damaging free radicals, and favours the production of GABA.

"Mitochondria are specifically designed to use fat for energy. When our mitochondria use fat as an energetic source, its toxic load is decreased, the expression of energy producing genes are increased, its energetic output is increased, and the load of inflammatory energetic-end-products is decreased.

The key of these miraculous healing effects relies on the fact that fat metabolism and its generation of ketone bodies (beta-hydroxybutyrate and acetoacetate) by the liver can only occur within the mitochondrion, leaving chemicals within the cell but outside the mitochondria readily available to stimulate powerful anti-inflammatory antioxidants. The status of our mitochondria is the ultimate key for optimal health and while it is true that some of us might need extra support in the form of nutritional supplementation to heal these much needed energy factories, the diet still remains the ultimate key for a proper balance."

9. Endurance Performance

If you are an endurance athlete, and you haven't looked into the benefits of ketosis and endurance performance you are potentially missing out on a massive edge over your competition.

The studies done on ketosis and endurance sports performance paint a pretty clear picture – it helps. One of the most detailed studies on fat utilisation and performance (compared to a standard carb diet) was named the FASTER study - the results found that those who were on a ketogenic type diet had more mitochondria than the control group, lower oxidative stress, lower lactate load and that the fat adapted and fuelled athletes could function off fat for a much higher intensity than the non-fat adapted counter parts.

10. Decreased Pain & Lowered Inflammation

Ketosis has been shown to have anti-inflammatory properties while also assisting with pain relief. Reducing glucose metabolism influences pain, so this could be one potential mechanism of action.

11. Stable Energy Levels

Anyone who has recently switched from a standard western diet to a ketogenic diet will soon notice how their energy levels are stable throughout the day. No mid-afternoon slumps, no cravings for instant sugar or caffeine hits.

Fat (and the ketones produced from fat) are a readily available source of fuel. Once someone is fat adapted and in ketosis, they will find they can easily go hours (even days) without food and not have drastic energy level swings.

12. Migraine Treatment

Many people who suffer from migraines have reported great results when switching from a conventional high carb diet to a ultra-low carb ketogenic diet.

Ketogenic diets (KD) ameliorates headache and reduces drug consumption in migraineurs, while the Standard diet is fully ineffective on migraine in a short term observation. Our findings support the role of KDs in migraine treatment.

13. Clean Burning Fuel for the Body

When a cell breakdowns glucose for fuel, it generates more reactive oxygen species compared to fat. These free radicals are neutralised by antioxidants. So skip the supplements, restrict carbohydrates, eat more fat and operate off clean burning ketones instead!

14. Easier to Fast

One of the best ways to get into a state of ketosis is through fasting. However, anyone who is eating a standard high carb diet will shudder at the thought of going 12 hours or longer without food.

Yet once you are fat adapted and you are in a state of nutritional ketosis, fasting becomes extremely easy.

15. Parkinson's Disease

Ketosis has also been shown to help those suffering from Parkinson's disease.

16. Epilepsy

The ketogenic diet has long been successfully used with those suffering from epilepsy. In fact, the ketogenic diet was first developed in 1921 to treat drug resistant epilepsy in children. Since then, numerous studies have been done showing how ketosis can help with epilepsy.

17. Cancer

Ketosis as a form of cancer treatment (and prevention) is rapidly growing in popularity. Why is that? Because so many cancer patients are reporting huge benefits when following a ketogenic diet. And why may that be? Many cancer cells can only survive with glucose as a fuel source.

By depriving a cancer cell of glucose by eating a ketogenic diet, we may be able to starve the cancer resulting in its death.

18. Acne

There is a lot of emerging evidence that ketosis can help clear acne. It has been shown that high glycemic foods can stimulate acne outbreaks and as the ketogenic diet goes without such foods it makes sense that acne should improve.

19. General Health

A ketogenic diet lead to:

Improved cholesterol levels

Decreased triglyceride levels

Decreased weight and fat mass

KETOGENIC DIET: BEGINNERS GUIDE

What is a Ketogenic Diet?

The ketogenic diet (often termed keto) is a very low-carb, high-fat diet that shares many similarities with the Atkins and low-carb diets.

It involves drastically reducing carbohydrate intake, and replacing it with fat. The reduction in carbs puts your body into a metabolic state called ketosis.

When this happens, your body becomes incredibly efficient at burning fat for energy. It also turns fat into ketones in the liver, which can supply energy for the brain.

Ketogenic diets can cause massive reductions in blood sugar and insulin levels. This, along with the increased ketones, has numerous health benefits.

Bottom Line: The ketogenic diet (keto) is a low-carb, high-fat diet. It lowers blood sugar and insulin levels, and shifts the body's metabolism away from carbs and towards fat and ketones.

Different Types of Ketogenic Diets

There are several versions of the ketogenic diet, including:

Standard ketogenic diet (SKD): This is a very low-carb, moderate-protein and high-fat diet. It typically contains 75% fat, 20% protein and only 5% carbs.

Cyclical ketogenic diet (CKD): This diet involves periods of higher-carb refeeds, such as 5 ketogenic days followed by 2 high-carb days.

Targeted ketogenic diet (TKD): This diet allows you to add carbs around workouts.

High-protein ketogenic diet: This is similar to a standard ketogenic diet, but includes more protein. The ratio is often 60% fat, 35% protein and 5% carbs.

However, only the standard and high-protein ketogenic diets have been studied extensively. Cyclical or targeted ketogenic diets are more advanced methods, and primarily used by bodybuilders or athletes.

Bottom Line: There are several versions of the ketogenic diet. The standard ketogenic diet (SKD) is the most researched and most recommended.

Ketogenic Diets Can Help You Lose Weight

A ketogenic diet is an effective way to lose weight and lower risk factors for disease. In fact, research shows that the ketogenic diet is far superior to the recommended low-fat diet.

What's more, the diet is so filling that you can lose weight without counting calories or tracking your food.

People on a ketogenic diet lost 2.2 times more weight than those on a calorie-restricted low-fat diet. Triglyceride and HDL cholesterol levels also improved.

There are several reasons why a ketogenic diet is superior to a low-fat diet. One is the increased protein intake, which provides numerous benefits.

The increased ketones, lowered blood sugar levels and improved insulin sensitivity may also play a key role.

Bottom Line: A ketogenic diet can help you lose much more weight than a low-fat diet. This often happens without hunger.

Ketogenic Diets for Diabetes and Prediabetes

Diabetes is characterized by changes in metabolism, high blood sugar and impaired insulin function.

The ketogenic diet can help you lose excess fat, which is closely linked to type 2 diabetes, prediabetes and metabolic syndrome. One study found that the ketogenic diet improved insulin sensitivity by a whopping 75%.

Bottom Line: The ketogenic diet can boost insulin sensitivity and cause fat loss, leading to drastic improvement for type 2 diabetes and prediabetes.

Other Health Benefits of the Ketogenic Diet

The ketogenic diet actually originated as a tool for treating neurological diseases, such as epilepsy.

Studies have now shown that the diet can have benefits for a wide variety of different health conditions:

Heart disease: The ketogenic diet can improve risk factors like body fat, HDL levels, blood pressure and blood sugar

Cancer: The diet is currently being used to treat several types of cancer and slow tumor.

Alzheimer's disease: The diet may reduce symptoms of Alzheimer's and slow down the disease's progression.

Bottom Line: A ketogenic diet may provide many health benefits, especially with metabolic, neurological or insulin-related diseases.

Foods to Avoid

In short, any food that is high in carbs should be limited.

Here is a list of foods that need to be reduced or eliminated on a ketogenic diet:

Sugary foods: Soda, fruit juice, smoothies, cake, ice cream, candy, etc.

Grains or starches: Wheat-based products, rice, pasta, cereal, etc.

Fruit: All fruit, except small portions of berries like strawberries.

Beans or legumes: Peas, kidney beans, lentils, chickpeas, etc.

Root vegetables and tubers: Potatoes, sweet potatoes, carrots, parsnips, etc.

Low-fat or diet products: These are highly processed and often high in carbs.

Some condiments or sauces: These often contain sugar and unhealthy fat.

Unhealthy fat: Limit your intake of processed vegetable oils, mayonnaise, etc.

Alcohol: Due to its carb content, many alcoholic beverages can throw you out of ketosis.

Sugar-free diet foods: These are often high in sugar alcohols, which can affect ketone levels in some cases. These foods also tend to be highly processed.

Bottom Line: Avoid carb-based foods like grains, sugars, legumes, rice, potatoes, candy, juice and even most fruits.

Foods to Eat

You should base the majority of your meals around these foods:

Meat: Red meat, steak, ham, sausage, bacon, chicken and turkey.

Fatty fish: Such as salmon, trout, tuna and mackerel.

Eggs: Look for pastured or omega-3 whole eggs.

Butter and cream: Look for grass-fed when possible.

Cheese: Unprocessed cheese (cheddar, goat, cream, blue or mozzarella).

Nuts and seeds: Almonds, walnuts, flaxseeds, pumpkin seeds, chia seeds, etc.

Healthy oils: Primarily extra virgin olive oil, coconut oil and avocado oil.

Avocados: Whole avocados or freshly made guacamole.

Low-carb veggies: Most green veggies, tomatoes, onions, peppers, etc.

Condiments: You can use salt, pepper and various healthy herbs and spices.

It is best to base your diet mostly on whole, single ingredient foods. Here is a list of 44 healthy low-carb foods.

Bottom Line: Base the majority of your diet on foods such as meat, fish, eggs, butter, nuts, healthy oils, avocados and plenty of low-carb veggies.

A Sample Ketogenic Meal Plan For 1 Week

To help get you started, here is a sample ketogenic diet meal plan for one week:

Monday

Breakfast: Bacon, eggs and tomatoes.

Lunch: Chicken salad with olive oil and feta cheese.

Dinner: Salmon with asparagus cooked in butter.

Tuesday

Breakfast: Egg, tomato, basil and goat cheese omelet.

Lunch: Almond milk, peanut butter, cocoa powder and stevia milkshake.

Dinner: Meatballs, cheddar cheese and vegetables.

Wednesday

Breakfast: A ketogenic milkshake (try this or this).

Lunch: Shrimp salad with olive oil and avocado.

Dinner: Pork chops with Parmesan cheese, broccoli and salad.

Thursday

Breakfast: Omelet with avocado, salsa, peppers, onion and spices.

Lunch: A handful of nuts and celery sticks with guacamole and salsa.

Dinner: Chicken stuffed with pesto and cream cheese, along with vegetables.

Friday

Breakfast: Sugar-free yogurt with peanut butter, cocoa powder and stevia.

Lunch: Beef stir-fry cooked in coconut oil with vegetables.

Dinner: Bun-less burger with bacon, egg and cheese.

Saturday

Breakfast: Ham and cheese omelet with vegetables.

Lunch: Ham and cheese slices with nuts.

Dinner: White fish, egg and spinach cooked in coconut oil.

Sunday

Breakfast: Fried eggs with bacon and mushrooms.

Lunch: Burger with salsa, cheese and guacamole.

Dinner: Steak and eggs with a side salad.

Always try to rotate the vegetables and meat over the long term, as each type provides different nutrients and health benefits.

Bottom Line: You can eat a wide variety of tasty and nutritious meals on a ketogenic diet.

Healthy Ketogenic Snacks

In case you get hungry between meals, here are some healthy, keto-approved snacks:

Fatty meat or fish.

Cheese.

A handful of nuts or seeds.

Cheese with olives.

1–2 hard-boiled eggs.

90% dark chocolate.

A low-carb milk shake with almond milk, cocoa powder and nut butter.

Full-fat yogurt mixed with nut butter and cocoa powder.

Strawberries and cream.

Celery with salsa and guacamole.

Smaller portions of leftover meals.

Bottom Line: Great snacks for a keto diet include pieces of meat, cheese, olives, boiled eggs, nuts and dark chocolate.

Tips for Eating Out on a Ketogenic Diet

It is not very hard to make most restaurant meals keto-friendly when eating out.

Most restaurants offer some kind of meat or fish-based dish. Order this, and replace any high-carb food with extra vegetables.

Egg-based meals are also a great option, such as an omelet or eggs and bacon.

Another favorite is bun-less burgers. You could also leave the bun and swap the fries for vegetables instead. Add extra avocado, cheese, bacon or eggs.

At Mexican restaurants, you can enjoy any type of meat with extra cheese, guacamole, salsa and sour cream.

For dessert, ask for a mixed cheese board or double cream with berries.

Bottom Line: When eating out, select a meat, fish or egg-based dish. Order extra veggies instead of carbs or starches, and have cheese for dessert.

Side Effects and How to Minimize Them

Although the ketogenic diet is safe for healthy people, there may be some initial side effects while your body adapts.

This is often referred to as "keto flu" – and is usually over within a few days.

Keto flu includes poor energy and mental function, increased hunger, sleep issues, nausea, digestive discomfort and decreased exercise performance.

In order to minimize this, you can try a regular low-carb diet for the first few weeks. This may teach your body to burn more fat before you completely eliminate carbs.

A ketogenic diet can also change the water and mineral balance of your body, so adding extra salt to your meals or taking mineral supplements can help.

For minerals, try taking 3,000–4,000 mg of sodium, 1,000 mg of potassium and 300 mg of magnesium per day to minimize side effects.

At least in the beginning, it is important to eat until fullness and to avoid restricting calories too much. Usually a ketogenic diet causes weight loss without intentional calorie restriction.

Bottom Line: Many of the side effects of starting a ketogenic diet can be limited. Easing into the diet and taking mineral supplements can help.

Supplements For a Ketogenic Diet

Although no supplement is necessary, some can be useful.

MCT oil: Added to drinks or yogurt, MCT oil provides energy and helps increase ketone levels.

Minerals: Added salt and other minerals can be important when starting out, due to shifts in water and mineral balance.

Caffeine: Caffeine can have benefits for energy, fat loss and performance.

Exogenous ketones: This supplement can help raise the body's ketone levels.

Creatine: Creatine provides numerous benefits for health and performance. This can help if you are combining a ketogenic diet with exercise.

Whey: Use half a scoop of whey protein in shakes or yogurt to increase your daily protein intake.

Bottom Line: Certain supplements can be beneficial on a ketogenic diet. These include exogenous ketones, MCT oil and minerals.

Frequently Asked Questions

Here are answers to some of the most common questions about the ketogenic diet.

1. Can I ever eat carbs again?

Yes. However, it is important to eliminate them initially. After the first 2–3 months, you can eat carbs on special occasions — just return to the diet immediately after.

2. Will I lose muscle?

There is a risk of losing some muscle on any diet. However, the high protein intake and high ketone levels may help minimize muscle loss, especially if you lift weights.

3. Can you build muscle on a ketogenic diet?

Yes, but it may not work as well as on a moderate-carb diet. More details: Low-Carb/Ketogenic Diets and Exercise Performance.

4. Do I need to refeed or carb load?

No. However, a few higher-calorie days may be beneficial every now and then.

5. How much protein can I eat?

Protein should be moderate, as a very high intake can spike insulin levels and lower ketones. Around 35% of total calorie intake is probably the upper limit.

6. What if I am constantly tired, weak or fatigued?

You may not be in full ketosis or be utilizing fats and ketones efficiently. To counter this, lower your carb intake and re-visit the points above. A supplement like MCT oil or ketones may also help.

7. My urine smells fruity? Why is this?

Don't be alarmed. This is simply due to the excretion of byproducts created during ketosis.

8. My breath smells. What can I do?

This is a common side effect. Try drinking naturally flavored water or chewing sugar-free gum.

9. I heard ketosis was extremely dangerous. Is this true?

People often confuse ketosis with ketoacidosis. The former is natural, while the latter only occurs in uncontrolled diabetes.

Ketoacidosis is dangerous, but the ketosis on a ketogenic diet is perfectly normal and healthy.

10. I have digestion issues and diarrhea. What can I do?

This common side effect usually passes after 3–4 weeks. If it persists, try eating more high-fiber veggies. Magnesium supplements can also help with constipation.

A Ketogenic Diet is Great, But Not For Everyone

A ketogenic diet can be great for people who are overweight, diabetic or looking to improve their metabolic health.

It may be less suitable for elite athletes or those wishing to add large amounts of muscle or weight.

And, as with any diet, it will only work if you are consistent and stick with it in the long-term.

That being said, few things are as well proven in nutrition as the powerful health and weight loss benefits of a ketogenic diet.

SUPPLEMENTS AND WORK-OUTS WHILST ON KETOGENIC DIET

Supplements Whilst On Ketogenic Diet

Why Supplement?

On any diet, supplementation is not a necessity, but beneficial. The same can be said for a ketogenic diet.

The reason for supplementing is often in order to maximise your intake of a certain macro/micronutrient if the diet requires you to eat a large quantity of it, or if it restricts certain foods, like carbohydrates, meaning you miss out on some key nutrients.

#1 Omega 3

Omega 3 is an essential fatty acid which is found from dietary sources of oily fish such as mackerel, salmon and sardines. It cannot be synthesised in the body; therefore, it must be taken in through our diets.

For many people, it is not possible to eat fish in such high quantities in order to receive the optimal levels of omega 3, as well as omega 6 and 9. Therefore, supplementing with omega 3 supplements such as fish oil is a great way to boost your intake.

There has also been research to suggest that fish oil supplements can lower levels of blood triglycerides. This is especially beneficial whilst on a ketogenic diet, since one of the risks when following it is that your levels of blood triglycerides may become too high.

By supplementing with omega 3 and fish oil supplements, you can help combat this and enjoy the benefits of the ketogenic diet, without worrying about any side effects.

#2 Coconut Oil

Coconut oil is an excellent 'supplement' which can be utilised for many different health benefits. coconut oil keto diet It is excellent for the ketogenic diet, since it can be used in order to boost your fat intake. What's more, its excellent for boosting your healthy fat intake.

Coconut oil is one of the only plant based fat sources which is saturated. This means if you want to get enough saturated fat in your diet, but do not want to have unhealthy, heavily processed fats, or animal fats, then coconut oil is a must.

You can purchase coconut oil in its raw form, which can be used for cooking, oil pulling, among others, or in the form of capsules, which might be more easy to take for someone who is just looking to increase their intake of healthy fats.

#3 Whey Protein

Possibly the most widely known and popular supplement out there. Whey protein is the most bio-available protein, and is quickly digested.

The reason you would take a whey protein supplement would be if you cannot get enough protein into your diet due to either cost, or because you need to minimise intake of other macronutrients.

Whilst on the ketogenic diet, since you are restricting where you get your calories from, it is a good idea to take protein supplements to ensure that you do not have to worry about consuming any carbs, or even fat from protein sources, meaning you have more room to play with elsewhere.

#4 Spirulina

Supplementing with greens such as spirulina is an excellent way of boosting the amount of vitamins and minerals you intake when following a ketogenic diet. spirulina-powder

What's more, spirulina is what is known as a complete protein, meaning that it contains all of the amino acids which your body needs in order to function properly.

Furthermore, spirulina contains moderate amounts of fibre. This makes it brilliant when following a ketogenic diet, since fibre helps to bind with carbohydrates and prevent them from being stored as fat.

#5 BCAAs

BCAAs, or branched chain amino acids, are a great supplement for all sorts of different individuals when following different diets.

One of the main benefits of BCAAs is to prevent muscle loss, especially when you are following a catabolic (tissue breakdown) meal plan. A ketogenic diet is just this, catabolic, since you are breaking down fat in order to lose weight. The issue is that you will lose some muscle. By supplementing with BCAAs, you can prevent your body from breaking down as much muscle as it normally would.

Furthermore, they can reduce the time it takes for your body to recover, which is vital when in a caloric deficit.

Conclusion

The ketogenic diet is an excellent diet for those who are looking to lose weight, especially those with a considerable amount to lose. These supplements will not only help you achieve your weight loss goals whilst following the ketogenic diet, but will improve your overall health and wellbeing.

Work-outs Whilst On Ketogenic Diets

Since going keto means greatly reducing carbs, and since carbs are the body's primary source of fuel, you might be wondering what your options are when it comes to how to exercise while in ketosis.

The good news is that while there are some things to keep in mind, exercise is totally possible on the ketogenic diet and even has some big benefits health- and energy-wise. These are important to know when wading through any misconceptions around low-carb eating and working out.

EXERCISING IN KETOSIS

First, let's note that the traditional view of weight loss—simply eating less and exercising longer, often with long bouts of cardio—is outdated and unsustainable. In order to see real results when it comes to losing weight and getting leaner, what you eat really matters. A great place to start is checking out a guide on sourcing meat, dairy, and seafood. Therefore, paying attention to the quality of your ketogenic diet itself, and maintaining a steady state of ketosis, is the most important first step you can take. To see if you are actually in a metabolic state of ketosis, testing your ketone levels is vitally important.

However, exercise also has many benefits for your health. It's good for the heart, builds muscle to keep you lean and toned, and strengths the bones. Thankfully, exercise can completely fit into your routine while eating for ketosis. You just need to keep in mind a few simple considerations:

TYPES OF EXERCISE

Nutritional needs vary depending on the type of exercise performed. Workouts styles are typically divided into four types: aerobic, anaerobic, flexibility, and stability.

Types of Exercise in Ketosis

Aerobic exercise, also known as cardio exercise, is anything that lasts over three minutes. Lower intensity, steady-state cardio is fat burning, making it very friendly for the keto dieter.

Anaerobic exercise is characterized by shorter bursts of energy, such as from weight training or high-intensity interval training. Carbohydrates are the primary fuel for anaerobic exercise, so fat alone can't provide enough energy for this type of workout.

Flexibility exercises are helpful for stretching out your muscle, supporting joints, and improving muscle range of motion. Increasing your flexibility can help prevent injuries caused by shortening of the muscles over time. Yoga and simple after-workout stretches are good examples of this.

Stability exercises include balance exercises and core training. They help improve your alignment, strength muscles, and control of movement.

When you're in ketosis, the workout intensity matters as well:

During low-intensity aerobic exercise, the body uses fat as its primary energy source.

During high-intensity aerobic exercise, carbohydrates are normally the main energy source.

30 KETOGENIC RECIPES

Avocado & Egg Fat Bombs, Deviled Eggs and Giveaway!

Ingredients

3 large cooked egg yolks

½ large avocado, peeled and seed removed (100 g/ 3.5 oz)

¼ cup mayonnaise (55 g/ 1.9 oz) - you can make your own

1 tbsp lemon or lime juice

½ tsp salt or to taste (I like pink Himalayan)

freshly ground black pepper

2 tbsp chopped spring onions or chives

Eat with:

freshly cut cucumber slices, bell peppers or crispy lettuce leaves

leftover cooked egg white halves (if making deviled eggs)

Discover foods, kitchen tools and other products I use and love! Find out more

Instructions

Start by cooking the eggs. Fill a small saucepan with water up to three quarters. Add a good pinch of salt. This will prevent the eggs from cracking. Bring to a boil. Using a spoon or hand, dip each egg in and out of the boiling water - be careful not to get burnt. This will prevent the egg from cracking as the temperature change won't be so sudden. To get the eggs hard-boiled, you need round 10 minutes. This timing works for large eggs. When done, remove from the heat and place in a bowl filled with cold water. I like and always use this egg timer! When the eggs are chilled, peel off the shells.

Halve the avocado and remove the seed and peel. Cut the eggs in half and carefully - without breaking the egg whites - spoon the egg yolks into a bowl

Place the avocado cut into pieces into a food processor and add the egg yolks, mayonnaise, lemon juice, salt and pepper. Process until smooth. Alternatively, mash with a fork until creamy and well combined.

Enjoy with cucumber slices and spring onion on top, or fill up the egg white halves and make deviled eggs. To avoid browning, store in an airtight container and keep for up to 5 days.

Keto Bread

Ingredients

1 1/2 Cup Almond Flour we get ours on amazon

6 Large eggs Separated

4 tbsp Butter melted

3 tsp Baking powder We use this!

1/4 tsp Cream of Tartar It's ok if you don't have this - We use this!

1 pinch salt

Servings:

20 Slices

Instructions

Preheat oven to 375.

Separate the egg whites from the yolks. Add Cream of Tartar to the whites and beat until soft peaks are achieved.

In a food processor combine the egg yolks, 1/3 of the beaten egg whites, melted butter, almond flour, baking powder and salt. Mix until combined. This will be a lumpy thick dough until the whites are added.

Add the remaining 2/3 of the egg whites and gently process until fully incorporated. Be careful not to overmix as this is what gives the bread it's volume!

Pour mixture into a buttered 8x4 loaf pan. Bake for 30 minutes. Check with a toothpick to ensure the bread is cooked through. Enjoy! 1 loaf makes 20 slices.

CAULIFLOWER CRUSTED GRILLED CHEESE SANDWICHES

INGREDIENTS:

1 head of cauliflower, cut into small florets and stem removed

1 large egg

1/2 cup shredded Parmesan cheese

1 tsp Italian herb seasoning

2 thick slices of white cheddar cheese

DIRECTIONS:

1. Preheat oven to 450F. Place cauliflower into food processor and pulse until crumbs about half the size of a grain of rice.

2. Place cauliflower into large microwave safe bowl and microwave for 2 minutes. Your cauliflower should be soft and tender (and hot!). (If you don't want to use the microwave to dry out the cauliflower and prefer to steam and wring with a cloth to dry, check out my wringing instructions here.)

3. Stir cauliflower to mix up the bottom and top cauliflower. Place back into the microwave and cook for another 3 minutes. Remove and stir again so that all the cauliflower cooks evenly. Place back into microwave and cook for 5 minutes. At this point, you should see the cauliflower is starting to become more dry. Microwave for another 5 minutes. Cauliflower should still be slightly moist to the touch, but should look dry and clumped up (like photo above; similar to as if someone had chewed it up and

spit it back out.) If you've made cauliflower pizza or breadsticks with the cloth wringing dry method, it should look the same.

4. Allow cauliflower to cool for a few minutes. Then add in egg, parmesan and seasoning. Stir to combine until smooth paste forms. Divide dough into 4 equal parts. Place onto large baking sheet lined with parchment paper or silpat mat. Using your knuckles and fingers, shape into square bread slices about 1/2 inch thick. Bake cauliflower bread for about 15-18 minutes or until golden brown. Remove from oven and let cool a few minutes.

5. Using a good spatula, carefully slide cauliflower bread off of parchment paper. Now you are ready to assemble your sandwiches. Normally I make grilled cheese sandwiches on a pan, but since the cauliflower crust is more delicate, I didn't want to risk it breaking with too many flips on the stove. Instead, make 2 cauliflower sandwiches by adding a slice of cheese in between each pair of bread slices. Place sandwiches into toaster oven and broil for several minutes (5-10) until cheese is completely melted and bread is toasty. If you don't own a toaster oven, you can also do this in the oven.

Chicken Pad Thai

Ingredients

⅛ teaspoon ground ginger

⅛ teaspoon garlic powder

⅛ teaspoon sea salt

⅛ teaspoon freshly ground black pepper

2 pounds free-range chicken tenders

2 tablespoons peanut oil

3 large free-range eggs, lightly beaten

⅓ cup organic chicken broth

3 tablespoons peanut butter

2 tablespoons tamari

1 tablespoon rice vinegar

½ cup chopped scallion

2 garlic cloves, minced

1 teaspoon red pepper flakes

4 zucchini, spiralized

½ cup bean sprouts

½ cup crushed peanuts, for garnish

1 lime, cut into wedges, for garnish

Instructions

In a medium bowl, mix the ginger, garlic powder, salt, and black pepper. Add the chicken tenders and toss until coated.

In a medium skillet, heat the peanut oil over medium-high heat. When the oil is hot, add the chicken tenders and cook, turning once, until cooked through, about 3 minutes. Remove the chicken from the skillet and cut into ¼-inch-thick slices. Set aside.

Add the eggs to the skillet and scramble them for about 1 minute. Remove the scrambled eggs from the skillet and set aside.

Reduce the heat under the skillet to medium-low and add the chicken broth, peanut butter, tamari, vinegar, scallion, garlic, and red pepper flakes. Stir well and cook for 3 minutes.

Add the chicken slices, zucchini noodles, scrambled eggs, and sprouts to the skillet. Toss to coat with the sauce, and cook for about 1 minute.

Serve the pad thai garnished with the peanuts and lime wedges.

7 Layer Spicy Taco Dip

Ingredients

1 (10 oz) container Sabra Supremely Spicy Hummus

2 cups guacamole

2 cups favorite chunky salsa

1½ cups plain Greek yogurt

2 Tbsp taco seasoning

1½ cups shredded Mexican cheese

1 cup diced roma tomatoes

½ cup sliced olives

¼ cup green onions, chopped

Instructions

In the bottom of an 8×8 or 7×11-inch baking dish, spread an even layer of hummus.

Top the hummus with a layer of guacamole, spreading evenly, then follow with a layer of salsa.

In a small bowl, mix together Greek yogurt with 2 tablespoons of taco seasoning until well combined and layer evenly on top of the salsa.

Sprinkle with shredded cheese followed by diced tomatoes, olives and green onions.

Serve with tortilla chips or veggies for dipping or cover and refrigerate until ready to serve.

Honey Curry Parsnip Fries

Ingredients

4 parsnips peeled and cut into quarters

3 tbsp olive oil

3 tbsp honey

2 tsp curry powder

salt and pepper to taste

parsley for garnish

Instructions

Pre-heat oven to 180c.

Place the peeled and quartered parsnips on a baking tray and drizzle with the olive oil and honey.

Toss to coat.

Add the curry powder and toss again.

Bake on the tray for about 20 minutes or until the parsnips are cooked through.

Leave to stand a minute or to. Letting them cool off slightly will result in a firmer fry.

Garnish the with parsley.

Crockpot Cheesy Bacon Chicken

Ingredients

Olive oil

3-5 chicken breast halves (just throw in whatever you need to feed your family. I thawed mine slightly just so I could slice them in chunks)

5 pieces cooked and crumbled bacon (I used turkey bacon that I cooked in the microwave)

¼ cup teriyaki sauce

½ cup Ranch salad dressing (hopefully you got some for cheap)

½ cup shredded cheddar cheese

Instructions

Pour about a tablespoon of olive oil the bottom of the crockpot. Place chicken in the crockpot.

In a small bowl mix together teriyaki sauce and ranch dressing (Yes, I know it seems weird... I was a little scared, but it is amazing!).

Pour over chicken. Toss crumbled bacon over top.

Cook on low for about 6 hours or on high for 3 hours. During the last 30 minutes, sprinkle the shredded cheese and allow to melt.

Brownie Fruit Pizza

Ingredients

1 package fudge brownie mix (8-inch square pan size)

1 package (8 ounces) cream cheese, softened

⅓ cup sugar

¾ cup crushed pineapple with juice

1 small banana, sliced

1 medium kiwifruit, peeled and sliced

1 cup sliced fresh strawberries

½ cup fresh blueberries

¼ cup fresh blackberries

¼ cup fresh raspberries

Instructions

Prepare brownie batter according to package directions. Spread batter out in a circle onto a greased pizza pan or cookie sheet (you can use a silpat liner instead). Bake at 375 degrees for 15-20 minutes or until a toothpick inserted near the center comes out clean. Cool completely.

In a large bowl, beat cream cheese and sugar until smooth.

Drain pineapple, reserving juice for later, and squeeze as much juice as you can out of pineapple. Add pineapple to the cream cheese mixture. Spread over brownie crust.

Toss banana slices in the pineapple juice; drain well. Arrange all the fruit on top of the cream cheese layer. Serve immediately or cover and refrigerate.

Strawberry Buttermilk Scones

Ingredients:

2 1/2 cups all-purpose flour

2 teaspoons baking powder

1 teaspoon baking soda

1/2 teaspoon fine sea salt

1/4 cup granulated white sugar

1/2 cup (1 stick) unsalted butter, very cold, cut into tablespoons

1 large Eggland's Best egg, cold

1/2 cup buttermilk, cold

1 cup fresh strawberries, hulled and diced

milk or cream, for brushing

Turbinado sugar or large crystal sugar, for sprinkling

Directions:

Preheat oven to 400°F. Line a baking sheet with parchment paper or silicone mat and set aside.

In a large bowl, whisk together the flour, baking powder, baking soda, salt, and sugar.

Add the cold butter. Cut into the flour mixture using a pastry blender, two forks, or your fingers until mixture resembles coarse sand.

In a small bowl, whisk together the egg and buttermilk. Pour into the dry mixture. Fold to combine. Midway through mixing, add the diced strawberries. Continue to fold until the strawberries are evenly distributed and the dough is mixed together.

Transfer the dough to a lightly floured surface. Pat the dough into a circle with a thickness of about 1-inch. Slice into 8 wedges.

Place the scones onto the prepared baking sheet, allowing at least 2 inch distance between scones. Lightly brush the top of each scone with heavy cream and sprinkle with turbinado sugar.

Bake for 20 to 25 minutes, until the scones have puffed up and the tops are lightly golden brown. Let the scones cool slightly on baking sheet before transferring to a wire rack. Serve warm or at room temperature.

Rye Tart Crust Recipe

Ingredients:

1 ½ cups all-purpose flour

½ cup rye flour

½ teaspoon kosher salt

12 tablespoons unsalted butter, chilled

1 egg yolk

¼ teaspoon cider vinegar

5 tablespoons ice water

Directions:

In the bowl of a stand mixer, combine the all-purpose flour, rye flour, and kosher salt. Turn on the stand mixer to low with the paddle attachment, and gradually add the butter, cut into small chunks. Mix until the dough is crumbly, with some small bits of butter chunks remaining. (If you don't have a stand mixer, place the flours and salt in a bowl and use a pastry cutter to cut in the butter.)

In a small bowl, mix several ice cubes and some water. In another bowl, combine the egg yolk, cider vinegar, and 5 tablespoons of the ice water, and whisk with a fork to combine. Turn the mixer on low and slowly pour the liquid mixture into the bowl until the dough comes together.

Remove the dough from the bowl and knead once or twice with your hands until the dough is smooth. Divide the dough into two even portions, form it into a disc, and wrap it in plastic wrap.

Allow to rest in the refrigerator for 30 minutes. If only using one dough, the other can be frozen in plastic wrap for later use.

Layered Buffalo Chicken Salad

Ingredients

2 cups shredded chicken

6 Tablespoons Frank's Buffalo Wing Sauce or GF wing sauce

½ (15 ounce) can black beans, rinsed and drained

3 cups butter lettuce, broken into small pieces

¼ cup blue cheese dressing

1 cup cheddar cheese, shredded

grape tomatoes, sliced

jalapeños, sliced

ripe avocado, diced and seasoned with salt

crumbled tortilla chips

Instructions

Shred chicken and mix with wing sauce. Spread chicken into an 8×8 casserole dish.

Sprinkle black beans on top. Add layer of cheddar cheese.

In separate bowl, toss lettuce with a light coat of blue cheese dressing then place on top of cheese.

Garnish with sliced tomatoes, jalapeños, avocado, and crushed tortilla chips.

Place in refrigerator for 1 hour to chill before serving.

Tri-Tip Sliders

Ingredients

2-3 pound Tri-Tip steak, using all the following ingredients for the rub; then cooked, cooled and sliced.

Rub Ingredients:

3 tablespoon Trader Joe's BBQ rub & seasoning with coffee and garlic

½ teaspoon lemon pepper

¼ teaspoon Montreal Steak Seasoning

½ teaspoon granulated garlic

1 teaspoon packed brown sugar

1 teaspoon salt

1 teaspoon garlic powder

1 teaspoon onion powder

For Caramelized Onions:

2 tablespoons butter

1 teaspoon garlic oil

2 medium yellow onions, halved and sliced paper thin (about 4 cups)

Kosher salt

Freshly ground black pepper

8 small slider rolls

1 bunch arugula, washed, dried, and torn

Sriracha Aioli Sauce

Instructions

Mix the rub ingredients together in a bowl. Place the roast in a baking pan with an edge because the rub is going to be sprinkled all over the meat, including the sides. Massage it into the meat. Cover and let sit at room temperature for an hour. Cook, cool and slice thin.

Melt the butter and oil in a large frying pan over medium-low heat until just foaming.

Add the onions and let them cook, stirring occasionally, until they are golden brown, about 40 minutes. Season with salt and pepper, remove from pan and let cool.

Toast the slider buns. Set oven to broil. Place slider buns on a baking sheet, separating the buns so that they are open-faced upwards. Broil until light and toasty only 1-2 minutes. Watch carefully!

Assemble the sliders by spreading the Sriracha Aioli Sauce on each bun, add Tri-Tip meat, then a few arugula leaves and some caramelized onions.

Crock pot Cinnamon Roll Casserole

Ingredients

2 cans of cinnamon rolls (any kind will do) – around 12 oz.

4 eggs

½ cup of milk

3 Tbsp maple syrup

2 tsp vanilla

1 tsp cinnamon

Instructions

Open up the cans of cinnamon rolls and set aside the icing for later.

Cut each cinnamon roll into quarters.

Spray your crock pot with non stick spray and place one of the rolls of cinnamon rolls in the bottom of the crock pot.

In a small bowl whisk together the eggs, milk, syrup, vanilla, and cinnamon.

Pour over the cinnamon rolls in the crock pot.

Place the remaining cinnamon rolls on top.

Drizzle one icing packet over the cinnamon rolls.

Place the crock pot lid on top and cook on low for 2 to 2½ hours.

Remove lid and drizzle the last icing packet over the cinnamon rolls.

Serve immediately and enjoy with a glass of milk!

Eggplant Rollatini

INGREDIENTS:

2 large eggplants, sliced lengthwise

½ teaspoon sea salt

½ teaspoon black pepper

1–1½ cups marinara sauce

2 large eggs

3 cups spinach

1 package goat feta (4 ounces)

1 teaspoon dried oregano

1 teaspoon parsley

1 teaspoon dried basil

2 cups pecorino romano, grated

1 cup raw sheep cheese, grated

DIRECTIONS:

Preheat oven to 450 F.

While your oven is heating up, cut the ends off of the two eggplants and then slice lengthwise.

Place the eggplant slices on a baking sheet lined with parchment paper and sprinkle with salt and pepper.

Bake for 12–15 minutes, remove and allow to cool.

Reduce heat to 400 F.

In a medium bowl, mix the eggs, goat cheese, spinach, oregano, parsley, basil, 1 cup pecorino romano, ½ cup raw sheep cheese, salt and pepper, mixing until well combined.

In a 9x13 baking dish, add ¾ cup marinara.

Place ¼ cup cheese mixture onto one end of the sliced eggplant, then roll it up and transfer to baking dish, continuing until baking dish is full.

Cover with remaining marinara and cheese.

Bake for 25 minutes and allow to cool for 10 minutes before serving.

Onion Soup

INGREDIENTS:

4 large onions, peeled and thinly sliced

2 cups chicken bone broth

2 cups beef bone broth

4 tablespoons ghee

5 garlic cloves, chopped

Sea salt and black pepper to taste

DIRECTIONS:

In a stock pot over medium heat, melt ghee and thinly sliced onions.

Cook onions until lightly caramelized.

Add bone broth and garlic.

Season with salt and pepper to taste.

Bring mixture to a boil and then reduce the heat and allow to simmer for 30–50 minutes (the longer, the more flavor).

Guiltless Garlic Parmesan Wings

INGREDIENTS:

12 chicken wings

1½ tablespoons avocado oil

1 tablespoon garlic powder

½ cup parmesan, grated

½ cup pecorino romano, grated

1 teaspoon salt

1 teaspoon pepper

DIRECTIONS:

Preheat oven to 350 F.

Line a baking sheet with parchment and set aside.

Mix spices and cheeses in a bowl.

Coat the wings in oil.

Dip wings in mixture.

Bake for 30 minutes.

Sweet Potato Hash Brown Casserole

INGREDIENTS:

2 sweet potatoes, cubed

1–2 tablespoons melted butter

1 white onion, chopped

1½ cups goat yogurt

½ cup goat feta

½ cup goat cheddar

1 teaspoon sea salt

1–2 teaspoons pepper

¼ cup chives, chopped

DIRECTIONS:

Preheat oven to 350 F.

In medium bowl, mix the onion, yogurt, goat cheddar and goat feta.

Add in sweet potatoes and melted butter.

Add mixture to baking dish.

Sprinkle extra goat cheddar on top.

Add sea salt, pepper and chives.

Bake for 55 minutes.

Olive Tapenade

INGREDIENTS:

1½–2 cups pitted black and green olives

¼–½ cup sun-dried tomatoes

½ cup capers, drained

½ teaspoon Himalayan pink salt

½ teaspoon pepper

½ teaspoon garlic

½ teaspoon onion powder

1½ teaspoon oregano

½ cup fresh basil leaves

½ cup fresh parsley leaves

2 tablespoons olive oil or avocado oil

DIRECTIONS:

Add everything to a food processor and blend on high until well combined.

Put on top of gluten-free crackers or toasted bread.

Jalapeño Poppers Recipe

INGREDIENTS:

10–12 jalapeño peppers, stemmed removed, sliced in ½ length-wise and seeds removed

1 package turkey bacon (optional*)

½-1 cup goat feta

½-1 cup shredded goat cheese

½ teaspoon cumin

½ teaspoon chili powder

½ teaspoon smoked paprika

½ teaspoon oregano

salt and pepper to taste

DIRECTIONS:

Preheat oven to 350 F.

Line a baking sheet, or two, with parchment paper and set aside.

In a medium-sized bowl add everything except the jalapeños and turkey bacon, mixing until well-combined.

Using your hands, fill each halved jalapeño with the cheese mixture.

Wrap jalapeño with turkey bacon and place on baking sheet.

Bake for 20 minutes.

Pair with our Avocado Ranch Dressing

Baba Ganoush Recipe

INGREDIENTS:

1 eggplant, sliced

1 cup tahini

3–4 garlic cloves, smashed

1–2 tablespoons avocado oil

1 cup parsley, chopped

Sea salt and pepper to taste

DIRECTIONS:

On a baking sheet lined with parchment paper, lay out the eggplant slices.

Salt the eggplant and allow eggplant to sit for 15–20 minutes to remove moisture.

Use a paper towel to dab eggplant, removing excess water.

Broil eggplant on top oven rack for 5–8 minutes.

Remove skin (optional*).

Place eggplant in a food processor and pulse until broken down.

Place all other ingredients in the food processor and blend on high until well combined.

Serve with chopped vegetables.

Spaghetti Squash Recipe

INGREDIENTS:

1 spaghetti squash

10 basil leaves, chiffonaded

1 cup sun-dried tomatoes, chopped

4 ounces sheep's feta, crumbled

Dressing:

2 tablespoons olive oil

2 tablespoons balsamic vinegar

sea salt and pepper, to taste

DIRECTIONS:

Preheat oven to 400 F.

Line a baking sheet with parchment paper and set aside.

Cut spaghetti squash in half length-wise and place face down on baking sheet.

Roast the squash for 20 minutes or until the flesh is easily pierced with a fork.

Scrape out spaghetti squash into a large bowl.

Top spaghetti squash with basil, sun-dried tomatoes and sheep's feta.

Whisk together olive oil, balsamic vinegar, sea salt and pepper and pour over spaghetti squash mixture.

Toss spaghetti salad mixture and serve while warm.

Steak Fajitas Recipe

INGREDIENTS:

1½ pounds skirt steak

1 green bell pepper, sliced

1 red bell pepper, sliced

1 red onion, sliced

1–2 jalapeños, sliced

1–2 cups salsa

Fajita Spice Blend

1 tablespoon chili powder

1 tablespoon oregano

1 tablespoon cumin

1 tablespoon garlic powder

½ tablespoon onion powder

1 teaspoon smoked paprika

1 teaspoon salt

1 teaspoon pepper

Toppings

massaged kale

plain goat yogurt

tomatoes, chopped

green onions, chopped

cilantro

DIRECTIONS:

Place everything into a crock pot and cook on low for 8 hours.

Serve on grain-free tortillas, topped with kale, plain goat yogurt, tomatoes, green onions and cilantro.

Summer Sautéed Veggies Recipe

INGREDIENTS:

1 tablespoon coconut oil

5 cloves garlic, sliced

2 yellow squash, halved and sliced

1 zucchini, halved and sliced

1 cup red grape tomatoes

½ teaspoon sea salt

½ teaspoon black pepper

2 tablespoons chopped fresh oregano

DIRECTIONS:

In a large skillet, heat oil over medium-high heat.

Add garlic and cook, stirring for about 30 seconds.

Add yellow squash, zucchini, salt and pepper. Stir and cook for about 3 minutes.

Stir in the red and yellow tomatoes and continue cooking just until vegetables are tender (about 3 more minutes).

Remove from heat and stir in the oregano

Raw Vegan Tomato Sauce Recipe

INGREDIENTS:

4 cups sundried tomatoes

5 cups Roma tomatoes

⅔ cup basil

4 cloves garlic, crushed

sea salt to taste

DIRECTIONS:

In a food processor, process all the ingredients, except for the sun-dried tomatoes. Gradually add in sun-dried tomatoes until a thick, smooth paste is formed.

Serve mixed in with zoodles topped with fresh basil or use as a dip with our garlic breadsticks!

Vegan Alfredo Recipe

INGREDIENTS:

1 small head of cauliflower, chopped (about 3 heaping cups)

2 tablespoons olive oil

2 cloves garlic, smashed and minced

2 teaspoons pine nuts

2¼ cup almond milk

2 teaspoons of each: salt, pepper, oregano and basil

juice of half a lemon

¼ cup plus 1 tablespoon nutritional yeast

DIRECTIONS:

In a medium-sized pot, cook the olive oil, garlic and pine nuts over medium heat for 3–4 minutes, or until garlic is golden brown.

Add in the almond milk and bring to a boil.

Reduce heat to medium and add the cauliflower and spices and cook until cauliflower is soft (about 8 minutes).

Transfer to a high-powered blender and add in the lemon juice and nutritional yeast and blend on high until smooth.

Add over your favorite gluten-free pasta or zoodles and top with fresh basil.

Wakame Pate Recipe

INGREDIENTS:

2 cups sunflower seeds, soaked for a minimum of 2 hours

1 teaspoon of each dried dulse seaweed and dried wakame

2 cloves garlic, crushed

½ lemon, juiced

½ teaspoon dill

2 tablespoons pickle brine

½ cup dill pickles, chopped

4 teaspoons minced red onion

½ cup minced celery

DIRECTIONS:

Combine sunflower seeds, dulse, garlic, lemon juice, dill and pickle brine in food processor and pulse until well combined (mixture will look like tuna salad).

Transfer to medium-sized mixing bowl, and fold in pickles, red onion and celery.

Serve cold and garnish with fresh dill and freshly ground black pepper to taste.

Served on flax crackers.

Cauliflower Fried Rice Recipe

INGREDIENTS:

1 medium head of cauliflower

4 tablespoons ghee

½ teaspoon garlic powder

½ teaspoon of each: sea salt and pepper

1 large carrot, shredded

1 medium onion, diced

4 eggs

¼ cup coconut aminos

DIRECTIONS:

Chop cauliflower into small florets and add to vitamix. Blend until consistency of rice pieces is achieved.

In a large skillet over medium heat, add 2 tablespoons ghee and cauliflower. Add garlic, salt, and pepper and cook for 5 minutes.

Add carrot and onion and cook until softened.

Add remaining ghee and eggs. Stir to scramble them and chop finely.

Stir in coconut aminos and serve.

Grain-Free Oatmeal Recipe

INGREDIENTS:

2 cups shredded coconut

½ –1 cup hemp seeds (less if you choose to add dried fruit to your base mix)

½ cup chia seeds

½ cup whole or coarsely ground flaxseeds

¼ teaspoon sea salt

OPTIONAL

½ cup chopped dried fruit

¼–½ teaspoon various spices. My favorite flavor combos are (1) cinnamon, cardamom, ginger; (2) cinnamon, cumin, cardamom, black pepper, coriander; (3) cloves, allspice, nutmeg, ginger, cinnamon; (4) rosemary, garlic, sage, cayenne

DIRECTIONS:

Combine all ingredients in a bowl and stir together thoroughly.

Include any optional ingredients you like.

Transfer to a wide-mouth quart jar to store in the refrigerator.

To prepare 1 serving of oatmeal, place 1/2 cup of dry mix in a bowl and add 1–1½ cups very hot water (just shy of boiling).

Stir well and allow to sit for 3–5 minutes.

Add fresh fruits, nuts, unsweetened chocolate, bacon crumbles, chicken or turkey sausage, coconut or almond milk, honey, coconut oil, or grass-fed butter to make it exciting.

Lamb Burgers Recipe

INGREDIENTS:

1 jalapeno, remove seeds sliced lengthwise

1/2 medium red onion, sliced

1 clove garlic, peeled

1 pound minced lean lamb

1 pound lean ground beef

1/2 cup small cubed raw aged sharp cheddar

1 tablespoon pink Himalayan salt

1/2 teaspoon ground cumin

1/2 teaspoon chili powder

1/4 teaspoon smoked paprika

1 teaspoon dried oregano

1/2 teaspoon coconut oil

DIRECTIONS:

In the bowl of a food processor, combine the jalapeno, onion and garlic and pulse until finely chopped.

Transfer the mixture to a large mixing bowl along with the lamb, ground beef, cheese and spices, using your hands to combine all the ingredients. Form 8 patties.

Chill in the refrigerator for 15–20 minutes to firm.

In a large nonstick skillet over medium-high heat, melt the coconut oil. Fry the burgers for 7–8 minutes per side, until firm to the touch and nicely browned.

Serve hot with your favorite toppings on a gluten-free bun, bed of lettuce or wrap in lettuce.

Cauliflower Tabbouleh Salad Recipe

INGREDIENTS:

1 large head cauliflower

½ cup lemon juice

¾ cup extra virgin olive oil

1 bunch parsley, washed and chopped

1 bunch green onions, chopped

2 cups Roma tomatoes, chopped

1 teaspoon salt

1 teaspoon pepper

DIRECTIONS:

Chop cauliflower then add to a food processor and pulse until rice-like consistency.

In a large bowl, combine the cauliflower and the lemon juice and stir well.

Add the olive oil and the parsley, green onions, tomatoes, salt and pepper.

Stir well.

Taste and add more salt and pepper if needed.

Cover and refrigerate for at least 4 hours, stirring once each hour.

Seared Grass-Fed Steak

INGREDIENTS:

2 steaks of grass-fed beef, your favorite cut, no more than 1–1/2 inches thick

salt and pepper

2 teaspoons avocado oil

DIRECTIONS:

Remove the steaks from the refrigerator, remove any packaging, and place in a baking dish. Allow the steaks to come to room temperature.

Heat the oven to 350 F.

Pat the steaks dry. Sprinkle the steaks with salt and pepper on both sides. Place the baking dish in the oven and bake the steaks for 10 minutes, flipping the steaks halfway through. With 2 minutes remaining on the timer, heat a skillet over medium-high heat.

Remove the steaks from the oven. Add the oil to the hot skillet and immediately add the steaks. Cook 2–4 minutes on each side, to your desired doneness, and sprinkle with more salt and pepper. Allow the steaks to rest for 5–8 minutes before serving.

Goat Cheese & Artichoke Dip Recipe

INGREDIENTS:

1 can artichoke hearts, drained

1 pound chevre goat cheese

2 tablespoons olive oil

2 teaspoons lemon juice

1 garlic clove, minced

½ cup pecorino, grated

1 tablespoons parsley

1 tablespoon chives

½ tablespoon basil

Sea salt and black pepper to taste

Dash of cayenne pepper

DIRECTIONS:

In a food processor, mix all ingredients except pecorino until well incorporated and creamy

Top with freshly grated pecorino

Baked Italian Chicken Recipe

INGREDIENTS:

4 chicken breasts

1 can of artichoke hearts, keeping a few out for garnishing the plate (optional)

1 cup mushrooms

1 onion, chopped

1 tomato, chopped

½ cup chicken stock

8 ounces of goat cheese chèvre

1 cup of spinach

garlic powder, salt, pepper and Italian seasoning, to taste

DIRECTIONS:

In a large skillet, cook the onions and mushrooms on medium-high heat until they are tender.

Remove from heat and place the onions and mushrooms in a bowl until you need them.

Using the same skillet, mix the goat cheese and the chicken stock together over medium heat. Stir until well mixed.

Add in the spices, tomatoes, artichokes, mushrooms, spinach and onions.

Cook until spinach is slightly wilted.

Place chicken breasts into the baking pan.

Pour veggie mixture over the chicken.

Bake the chicken at 350⁰ Fahrenheit for 30 minutes, or until done.

Gluten-Free Cauliflower Mac and Cheese Recipe

INGREDIENTS:

1 large cauliflower head, cut into small florets

½-¾ cup kefir

½ cup goat's milk cottage cheese, pureed

1½ tsp Dijon mustard

1½ cups grated sheep's or goat's milk cheddar cheese, plus additional for topping

½ teaspoon Black Pepper

1 teaspoon Sea Salt

⅛ teaspoon garlic powder

ghee

DIRECTIONS:

Preheat oven to 375 degrees Fahrenheit. Grease 8" x 8" pan with ghee.

Bring a pot of salted water to a boil. Add cauliflower and cook until slightly tender, about 5 minutes. Drain and pat dry with paper towels. Spread in prepared pan.

In a saucepan over medium-high heat, mix together kefir, cottage cheese, and mustard until smooth.

In a saucepan over medium high heat, mix together the cottage cheese, kefir and mustard until smooth

Stir in cheese, sea salt, black pepper, and garlic powder until cheese just starts to melt. Pour over cauliflower and stir. Top with additional cheese if desired and bake for 10–15 minutes.

Creamy Cucumber Avocado Soup Recipe

INGREDIENTS:

½ cucumber, peeled

1 ripe avocado

5 stalks celery

3 tablespoons lemon juice

¼-½ cup water

1 teaspoon sea salt

½ teaspoon black pepper

2 ounces raw cheddar cheese or goat cheese

DIRECTIONS:

Blend all ingredients (except the cheese) together in a high powered blender.

Serve chilled with cheese.

Chicken Vegetable Soup Recipe

INGREDIENTS:

3–4 carrots, peeled

1 onion, chopped

3–4 celery stalks, chopped

1 zucchini, thinly sliced

3 organic chicken breasts

5 cups chicken broth

sea salt and black pepper to taste

2 ounces raw cheese

DIRECTIONS:

Dice the chicken and chop the carrots, celery, zucchini and onion.

Place the chicken and vegetables in a large soup pot and cover with cold water. Heat and simmer, uncovered, until chicken is throughly cooked (usually over 30 minutes).

Strain the chicken and vegetables, then add them back into the pot. Pour in the broth, season with sea salt and black pepper, and heat up for 10 minutes. Top with cheese and serve.

Cheesy Bread Recipe

INGREDIENTS:

8 eggs

¾ cup water

1 cup kefir

1 teaspoon sea salt and ground black pepper

4 cups almond flour

1½ cups chia seeds

2 cups of shredded raw cheese

DIRECTIONS:

Preheat oven to 350 degrees F.

Whisk eggs, kefir, water, salt and pepper.

Add flour, chia and raw cheese to the mixture.

Pour into a greased loaf pan.

Bake for 40-45 minutes.

Roasted Red Pepper Sauce with Chicken Recipe

INGREDIENTS:

4 boneless, skinless organic chicken breasts

4 slices raw cheddar cheese

1 red bell pepper

¼ cup coconut oil

2 garlic cloves, minced

½ teaspoon onion powder

¼ teaspoon cayenne pepper

½ teaspoon sea salt

½ teaspoon thyme

DIRECTIONS:

Preheat oven to 500 degrees F.

Line a baking sheet with foil.

Remove the stem and seeds and cut bell pepper into medium size strips and place on the prepared baking sheet.

Drizzle with coconut oil and bake in oven for 10 minutes.

Place peppers in blender along with garlic cloves, onion powder, cayenne pepper, sea salt, and thyme. Blend until smooth.

Sauté chicken with coconut oil in a skillet and season with salt and pepper until chicken is cooked through.

Place cheese on each chicken breast, return to skillet and cover until cheese melts. Spoon a few tablespoons of red pepper sauce over chicken.

CONCLUSION

A ketogenic diet (keto) is a very low-carb diet, which turns the body into a fat-burning machine. It has many potential benefits for weight loss, health and performance, but also some potential initial side effects.

A ketogenic diet is similar to other strict low-carb diets, like the Atkins diet or LCHF (low carb, high fat). These diets often end up being ketogenic more or less by accident. The main difference between strict LCHF and keto is that protein is restricted in the latter.

With the right ketogenic diet plan you can turn your body into a fat burning machine, helping you increase your lean muscle and also helping you reduce that fat storage that is keeping you from obtaining your dream shape.

www.ingramcontent.com/pod-product-compliance
Lightning Source LLC
Chambersburg PA
CBHW062343280526
45787CB00012B/712